DEATH
CAN
WAIT

How I Beat Stage IV Cancer Naturally

WILLIAM HUDSON

Published by Holistic Healing Press

ISBN (paperback): 979-8-218-40383-6
ISBN (ebook): 979-8-218-40384-3

Book design and production by www.AuthorSuccess.com
Interior images from www.dreamstime.com

Printed in the United States of America

DEATH CAN WAIT

Dear reader, I want to express my admiration for your bravery and perseverance in picking up this book. Your decision is a testament to your commitment to yourself and your health. May the words within these pages give you the knowledge to make informed decisions about your health options. This book is dedicated to you and to my spiritual guides and teachers who inspired me to write it.

FREE BONUS CHAPTER OFFER

On my website is a free 'bonus chapter' for all subscribers on a little-known supplement that purportedly can reverse the biological aging process and help the body heal itself of whatever ails it holistically. You can get it here: https://williamhudson.org/nano-soma

Contents

Foreword

I had the privilege to read *Death Can Wait: How I Beat Stage IV Cancer Naturally.*

First, I love reading people's success stories, especially when it comes to health. Second, I am all for natural remedies and helping our bodies to heal themselves as they were intended to.

Working in emergency rooms for the past thirteen years has made me realize that we rely on medical science way too much without asking questions about medications, and their ability to treat and cure. It seems that for all ailments, there is always a pill or pills as an answer. If the drugs have side effects, then there's another prescription to address the issue. The more I've worked in the fast-paced ERs, the more I have realized that we keep treating, not curing. We're also sending the wrong message by prescribing medicines that help mask the symptoms without addressing the cause. We're enabling people to use medications as an excuse to continue with their unhealthy habits. Think about the diabetics who take their medicine and then indulge in sodas and sweets thinking that the disease has no more effect on them. We often fail people by not talking about the importance of balance in their lifestyle and daily habits. I have cared for countless patients with numerous comorbidities (diseases), only to be diagnosed with yet another disease, or the worst of all: cancer. Cancer has a dreaded sound to its name. Many of us think it rhymes with death. Indeed, it is a very scary word.

I have a collection of books on cancer as a metabolic disease and the result of cell respiration gone wrong. So, I was interested to read about William's personal journey to reach a cancer-free diagnosis. There is a recurring theme: the healing properties of naturally fermented food. Thank you, William, for sharing the easy-to-follow recipe!

A nice touch of his book is its simplicity. It is easy to read and follow, and straight to the point. He has no intention to bore you with fillers and side stories. He offers a simple and affordable direction to achieve a cancer-free life. There are numerous books, podcasts, lectures, and videos on cancer treatments. Often, they might appear confusing by only discussing parts of the disease-curing process. However, William was able to pull the most important components together by touching on diet, physical activity, mindfulness, and natural remedies.

He wants all of us to thrive in our health journey. This stems from a selfless, humble, and grateful perspective. Without health in our mind, body, and spirit, there is nothing.

Happy reading to you all!

Antonia McNamara APRN
(Advanced Practice Registered Nurse)

Introduction

From the moment of my diagnosis of stage IV metastatic melanoma in 2018, my life became a whirlwind.

During a regular checkup with my primary care physician, during an ordinary medical scan undertaken for an unrelated concern, they found an anomaly on my lower right lung. A biopsy confirmed it was stage IV metastatic melanoma. Suddenly, I found myself in a world I had only heard about—the world of "cancer."

My insurance company assigned me a pair of hospice workers who, almost immediately after the diagnosis, came to my home to speak with me and my husband. They offered to help with what they believed would be future medical appointments and keep me as least stressed as possible. They made sure we had all our financial and medical papers in order. They were expecting, as my doctors were, that I would get very sick and then die.

They were wrong.

My doctors wasted no time, advising immediate surgery to remove the melanoma in my right lung. After the operation, they initiated immunotherapy with OPDIVO, but I had an autoimmune response, forcing them to discontinue the treatment. (An autoimmune response is the immune system's misguided attack on the body's healthy cells and tissues, leading to various autoimmune diseases.) Physically, I felt fine. I didn't feel any pain, but there was stuff showing up in the scans of my lungs, and the doctors concluded it wasn't necessarily cancer but an autoimmune response, which sometimes happens with immunotherapy drugs. I have heard about many cancer patients, especially with melanoma, having great results with immunotherapy, so I would encourage you to explore this option with your oncologist. For me, it was a no-go, I think, because of my history of having autoimmune reactions to flu shots and other substances.

My oncologist and I agreed to pause all treatments at this time, awaiting the following scan results to determine if the cancer had spread.

Even after doing everything that my doctors had recommended, they still had something terrible to tell me. With my husband at my side, we confronted the grim prognosis given by my doctors. They said I probably only had eight to ten months to live. They urged me to "get my affairs in order" and "live life to its fullest." I felt vulnerable and afraid.

It was at this point that I made the decision: **I would not give up on myself**.

Ever.

With the words "get your affairs in order" echoing in my mind and beginning my research, I started to have reservations about entrusting my fate solely to conventional medicine. I realized that cancer was both a health concern *and* a multi-billion-dollar industry. I questioned whether the interests of patients always aligned with the interests of this mammoth medical industry. A lingering doubt nagged at me: could there be alternative solutions, options that existed beyond the cancer industry's purview?

This book is about how a path I never chose led me to the crossroads of choice. As I researched the possibilities of holistic healing, I understood that my body was not a battleground but a sacred vessel capable of healing itself when nurtured correctly. I soon **went from the fear of imminent death to the realization that I did not have to die (yet).** It is now more than six years after my diagnosis, and I remain cancer-free.

My research found that there were several alternative solutions to healing from cancer. Some were very expensive and required travel abroad and weeks away from home. Most were not covered by traditional medical insurance. I couldn't afford the more costly alternatives, leading me to two natural, simple solutions that didn't cost much. Determined to live, I started on this dual-pronged approach, and the results speak for themselves.

I believe everything happens for a reason. My diagnosis with "terminal" cancer became an opportunity for me to delve into extensive research and discover effective alternative cancer treatments and then be able to share them with you!

The alternative cancer treatments I cover in this book have been around for up to a century and have proven effective for thousands of patients. You'll hear testimonies from some of them.

What to Expect in the Pages Ahead

I ordered the chapters in this book according to their importance on what you can and should do to help heal yourself of cancer.

In Chapter 1, I address the emotional impact a cancer diagnosis had on me and talk about the whirlwind and the overwhelm I faced and how I confronted it.

Chapter 2 introduces a powerful way to start your cancer-healing journey. It explains how combining two simple food ingredients can promote cell bio-oxygenation and help reverse cancer cell growth.

In **Chapter 3**, I discuss a century-old holistic cancer clinic that has successfully treated patients that mainstream medicine has given up on. I explore its history, natural formula, and affordability of the treatments.

In **Chapter 4**, I explain how fluoride ended up in our water supply without the public understanding all the facts about its dangers. I also discuss the importance of chlorine in municipal water supplies and highlight the necessity of removing it from your drinking water. I provide safe methods of removing both fluoride and chlorine from your water.

In **Chapter 5**, I review when chemotherapy, according to at least one doctor, may or may not be appropriate for certain types of cancer. I also discuss the side effects of chemotherapy, and I address the question of whether chemotherapy can cause certain cancers to spread/metastasize.

Chapter 6 highlights the importance of taking digestive enzymes with every meal and supplementing your diet with probiotics daily. I also explore whether adopting a vegan diet could be beneficial for your situation and investigate the possible link between cancer and root canals. The chapter provides several other crucial considerations that can help you to make informed decisions about your health.

What You Will Take Away from This Book

Hope for a bright and healthy future.

Encouragement to move forward with simple steps to help you recover from cancer.

Confidence that you can do this!

Peace of mind, knowing that you are taking steps in the right direction for your life and health.

A sense of belonging to a **community** of others on a similar journey.

Ideas on things you can do to bring yourself to optimal health.

This is the journey of how I naturally and affordably conquered stage IV cancer. I wrote this book to give you **hope** and to let you know that you may be able to conquer cancer, as well.

If your doctors are still with you, please continue to work with them to make informed decisions. But if you want to learn about natural, affordable options to help increase your chances of surviving cancer, read on.

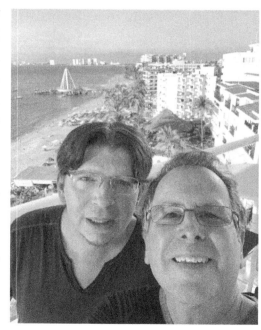

William and his husband Raymond vacationing in Puerto Vallarta, Mexico one month before his cancer diagnosis

CHAPTER 1

The Personal Impact of
a Cancer Diagnosis

Thinking back to when I was first diagnosed with cancer is difficult for me. Often, I have difficulty allowing my emotions to rise to the surface. I'm very left-brained: I tend to be logical and analytical instead of emotional and creative, as right-brained people are. I was, after all, drawn to a career in technology and in a higher education industry (thus very academic and left-brained).

Don't get me wrong, I have my right-brained moments: I'll cry during a good movie or when I think of a beloved pet dying. And I often shed a tear when I tell people about my cancer story.

A cancer diagnosis for most people, second to a loved one dying, has to be one of the most fearful and horrible things that can happen to a person! Thinking back, I suppose I may have been in shock? My initial diagnosis was stage IV, which, as opposed to, say, a stage I diagnosis, left me little time to contemplate my next steps. Stage IV, to most people, equals a death sentence. I was afraid. From my initial diagnosis to surgery, immunotherapy, then stopping immunotherapy was several months, but I remember it like it was only days. I felt numb.

A stage IV diagnosis can also leave little room for hope, but I had some. I already knew, for instance, that mainstream medicine only allowed for mainstream treatments, and most did not approve or condone holistic or natural healing outside of their modalities. However, I knew holistic treatments existed and was determined to find them. This understanding gave my left-brain self a project to work on—finding alternative solutions. Finding these solutions gave me hope. It also kept me busy and helped me from becoming overwhelmed by the emotions that would come naturally for anyone with a cancer diagnosis.

My diagnosis was in January of 2018, I had surgery in April, and I had already scheduled my first consultation at the holistic treatment center in November of that year, which gave me hope and something to look forward to.

Whether you are left-brained like me or right-brained like my husband, experiencing fear and many other emotions when facing a cancer diagnosis is normal.

It's crucial to recognize the emotional turbulence that comes with a cancer diagnosis. The uncertainty and fear of an unforeseeable future can be overwhelming. We might struggle with the injustice of the situation, and the emotional agony can even take a physical toll, further complicating things.

You probably already know this, but I want to gently remind you that it's okay to feel the emotions that come up for you. You may want to seek support from loved ones or professionals who can offer understanding and compassion. Allow yourself the space to feel what comes up and to find moments of comfort. You might try journaling, spending time in nature, or connecting with others who have faced a diagnosis. What's important to remember is that **you are not in this alone!**

There is a time to feel and express your emotions, and there is a time to take action. This book provides hope and practical steps that you can take to overcome cancer, even if your doctors have given up on you, as mine did. As you read this book and take steps towards healing, you may experience a range of emotions—excitement about the possibilities, hope for a healthy future, encouragement to take positive action, and love and compassion towards yourself and others in this community of people who are taking steps towards cancer healing.

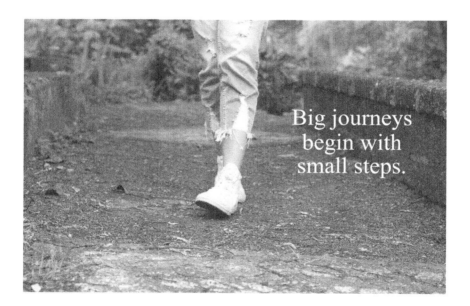

Big journeys begin with small steps.

CHAPTER 2

The Diet

This chapter covers a quick and affordable way to jumpstart your healing process from home. It's important to have quick wins and take immediate action steps to stay encouraged and continue moving in the right direction. In this chapter, we will delve into the **Budwig Diet**, an excellent example of a healing method that is both accessible and cost-effective.

The Budwig Diet: A Legacy of Healing

Dr. Johanna Budwig, a German biochemist and physicist born in 1908, created the Budwig Diet. She devoted her life to studying the relationship between diet and health, focusing on cancer. Her research revolved around the properties of essential fatty acids and their effects on cellular health.

Dr. Budwig conducted research in nutrition during a time when the scientific community was only starting to understand the importance of essential fatty acids, particularly omega-3s in flaxseed oil. Her groundbreaking research led her to a significant discovery: the beneficial effects of combining flaxseed oil with probiotic-infused cottage cheese.

According to the "Wellness Cancer Guide" provided by the Budwig Center in Malaga, Spain,[1] Dr. Budwig's method can help fight cancer by promoting bio-oxygenation. This is done by combining flaxseed oil with quark or cottage cheese. Dr. Budwig observed that cancer patients had an unusual greenish-yellow substance replacing the normal red oxygen-carrying hemoglobin, leading to weakness and anemia. She discovered that incorporating flaxseed oil and cottage cheese into the diet while eliminating harmful hydrogenated fats replaced abnormal blood elements with healthy red blood cells, alleviating weakness and anemia. In many cases, this led to the disappearance of cancer symptoms, liver dysfunction, and diabetes.

Blending and consuming them together is crucial to benefit from flaxseed oil and cottage cheese (or quark). The combination is synergistic, meaning that one ingredient's healthful properties trigger those of the other. Even cottage cheese that lacks probiotics loses its dairy properties, such as casein and lactose, when mixed with flaxseed oil. I am lactose intolerant, but I have had no issues with this mixture.

Dr. Budwig advised against using artificial, forced oxygen as an anti-cancer therapy. According to her, it is more important to maintain low oxygen levels within mitochondria rather than high levels. Oxygen therapies are discouraged because, in the context of cancer, the defective cells hinder correct oxygen utilization due to unhealthy fats in the Western diet. Increased atmospheric oxygen does not benefit cancer patients, as the cancerous condition disrupts the cells' ability to use oxygen effectively.

According to Dr. Budwig, the Budwig Protocol addresses this issue by restoring the cells' ability to breathe, allowing inhaled oxygen to function as intended.

"The most successful anti-cancer diet in the world."

Dr. Dan C. Roehm, MD, FACP, an oncologist and former cardiologist, wrote in a 1990 article published in the *Townsend Letter for Doctors and Patients* that Dr. Budwig's dietary approach showed unparalleled effectiveness as an anti-cancer regimen. Despite initial skepticism, Dr. Roehm attests, based on his extensive professional experience, that Dr. Budwig has convincingly demonstrated the high treatability of cancer. The key lies in making dietary and lifestyle changes, which yield an immediate response. In 1951, Dr. Budwig identified the precise biochemical breaking point in cancer cells, which can be corrected in vitro (in a test tube) and in vivo (in a living organism).

Dr. Roehm commends the remarkable construction of this diet and wishes that his patients had a deep understanding of biochemistry and quantum physics so they could better understand how amazing this diet is.

Dr. Roehm cited a 1967 interview on the South German Radio Network where Dr. Budwig stated that about 90 percent of patients could achieve health restoration within a few months, even in cases where surgery and radiation therapy had failed. Despite the lack of opposition to this remarkable news, it has not been widely communicated to people in this country.

Once the methodology is grasped, Dr. Roehm depicts the understanding of cancer treatment as straightforward and highly effective. However, he notes a desire among those with a vested interest in the cancer industry to conceal this information.

Dr. Dan C. Roehm extends a call for forgiveness to those who have suffered from this disease, along with their families and friends, urging understanding for those who have withheld this straightforward yet crucial information for so long.

Henderson and Garcia, in their book *Cancer-Free: Your Guide to Gentle, Non-toxic Healing*,[2] point out that Dr. Budwig's 90 percent success figure does not include chemotherapy recipients and recommend: "Don't lower your odds by submitting to chemotherapy."

Before discussing the diet, let's first look at the benefits of the two main ingredients: flax oil and probiotic-infused cottage cheese.

Omega-3 Rich Flaxseed Oil: Your Health Ally

Flaxseed oil is an excellent source of essential omega-3 fatty acids, especially ALA, which offer numerous health benefits. Omega-3s help promote heart health, aid cognitive function, and reduce inflammation. They help lower blood pressure, reduce triglyceride levels, and enhance overall cardiovascular function, reducing the risk of heart disease. People with chronic inflammation conditions like arthritis can benefit from the oil's anti-inflammatory properties, which alleviate joint pain and stiffness. Flax oil's omega-3s also help maintain skin health by reducing inflammation and maintaining moisture. They positively influence brain health, enhancing memory and cognitive performance. The oil's fiber content also supports healthy digestion and regular bowel movements. Lignan compounds in the oil may provide hormonal balance benefits, particularly for women experiencing menopausal symptoms. Lastly, research suggests that flaxseed oil consumption may significantly reduce LDL (harmful) cholesterol levels, emphasizing its positive impact on overall health.

The Power of Probiotic-Infused Cottage Cheese

This dairy product contains healthy probiotics that help maintain a balanced gut microbiome. The live cultures in probiotic-infused cottage cheese can create a diverse and healthy bacterial environment in your digestive system, improving digestion and nutrient absorption, reducing digestive discomfort, and providing better bowel regularity. Moreover, consuming this probiotic-rich cottage cheese may also help boost your immune system, as a significant portion of your immune function is related to your gut health.

The Magic of the Budwig Formula

Clearly, the two primary components of the Budwig Diet offer numerous benefits. However, when utilized in conjunction, they create a potent blend that can facilitate healing on various levels. This harmonious combination generates a potent elixir that promotes cellular health.

If you want to try the Budwig Diet as part of your healing journey and have the resources to learn more about it, consider visiting the Budwig Center in Malaga, Spain. This way, you can fully immerse yourself in an environment dedicated to this approach and gain access to resources that can help guide you more precisely. However, if you are on a budget, you can still try this approach from home, like I did.

At a minimum, I recommend visiting their website, where you can find the official recipe for the "Budwig Mix" (as it is also called). I must confess that I don't follow this recipe to the letter. In this book, I'm sharing what I believe worked for me in preventing cancer from returning to my body. I've chosen to keep things simple and affordable by using only the two main ingredients, cottage cheese and flaxseed oil, combined in the proper proportions.

However, if you prefer to follow Dr. Budwig's original recipe strictly, the Budwig Center's website provides detailed instructions. Also, I urge caution when searching the internet for "Budwig diet," as you may encounter recipe variations that deviate from Dr. Johanna Budwig's original recipe.

The proper combination for the recipe is a two-to-one ratio of Nancy's probiotic low-fat cottage cheese to Barlean's flax oil (organic, pure, unrefined, and fresh cold-pressed). The Budwig Center recommends six tablespoons of cottage cheese to three tablespoons of flax oil. Some practitioners recommend a ratio of ten tablespoons of cottage cheese to five tablespoons of flax oil (which is what I did to start). Without cancer, I've transitioned back to the Center's recommended dosage of six tablespoons of cottage cheese to three tablespoons of flax oil. Blend until you reach a smooth consistency like whipped cream.

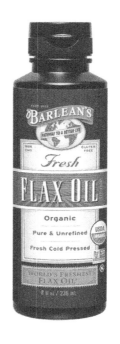

Please compare the recommendations of the Budwig Center with mine. I have the formula daily for breakfast and then eat normally for the rest of the day. However, it is important to be mindful of what you eat throughout

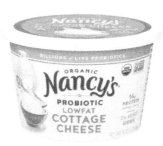

the day, as you will see in other parts of this book.

Unfortunately, the Budwig Diet has not received widespread support from mainstream medical practitioners. But I understand why. It's natural, can't be profited from by big pharma, and doctors who recommend it might lose their medical license.

Prominent doctors who have spoken favorably about the Budwig Diet and similar natural approaches to health include Dr. Andrew Weil, a well-known integrative medicine expert, and Dr. Nicholas Gonzalez, a holistic cancer treatment specialist. These doctors have explored various complementary and alternative therapies, including dietary approaches like the Budwig Diet, as part of a holistic approach to health and healing.

The Blender

I have found that using a reliable hand blender is essential when creating the Budwig Mix in my daily routine. I specifically use the Vitamix immersion blender as it has proven to be the best blender for me. Unfortunately, I have had the unpleasant experience of cheaper blenders breaking within months of daily use.

Reach out to Barlean's, the producer of the flax oil, and have it shipped to you. They offer a significant "cancer discount" for the flax oil, which can ease the financial burden. You can find more information and place orders by calling them at 800-445-3529.

It's worth noting that the availability of specific ingredients may vary depending on your location. If you encounter challenges in sourcing the exact ingredients for the Budwig Mix, the Budwig Center's website, mentioned earlier, provides valuable information on suitable substitutes. For example, if you can't find Nancy's brand of cottage cheese and use a different brand, I've found that it doesn't mix as well. Their website recommends mixing in low-fat milk to make the mix more consistent.

Testimonials paraphrased from Budwig Center website:[3]

In 2013, **Colleen M.** shared the story of her dog's battle with bone cancer, describing it as an aggressive form with a grim prognosis. The veterinarian had predicted that her dog would succumb to the illness within four weeks. Two weeks into the diagnosis, the dog's condition had deteriorated significantly; he was becoming emaciated, and Colleen had to bring his food and water to him. The dog had a noticeable cluster on his leg, rendering him unable to walk. X-rays revealed a dark spot in the bone with barely any bone left.

Having already experienced success with the Budwig protocol for her own health issues, including breast cancer and stage IV cirrhosis of the liver, Colleen wondered if the same approach could help her dog manage pain in his final days. Despite the dog's initial refusal, Colleen added a bit of Stevia to the Budwig Mix, and the dog enthusiastically consumed the entire bowl. To her surprise, the dog, who had not walked for days, eventually got up, limped, and indicated a desire to go outside. Over the following days, the dog's condition improved steadily.

Six weeks from the initial cancer diagnosis and four weeks into the Budwig protocol, the previously observed cluster had disappeared, the dog had regained all lost weight, resumed walking, and exhibited overall improved functionality. Colleen marveled at the remarkable transformation and considered the experience truly amazing.

Since December 2011, **Valerie K.** has been incorporating a regimen of six UK dessert spoons of flax oil with cottage cheese as part of her approach to combat breast metastases in the liver, lung, and lymph glands. Notably, all tumors and lymph glands have significantly reduced, and Valerie reports a continuous improvement in her overall well-being. It's noteworthy that Valerie has opted for a treatment plan excluding chemotherapy or radiation, relying solely on vitamins and other interventions.

Sandy B. shared that she initiated the cottage cheese and flaxseed oil protocol (and more) for colorectal Squamous Cell Carcinoma a year ago. Remarkably, doctors are currently puzzled as there seems to be no evidence of cancer in her condition.

Several years ago, **John** received treatment for a high fever in the emergency room, leading to a subsequent colonoscopy that revealed ulcerative colitis, bleeding ulcers in the duodenum, erythematous patches in his colon, and polyps removed through electro-snare cautery. Following the surgery, he experienced intense pain and cramping for several weeks. Transitioning to the Budwig protocol, John noticed improvement within two weeks, and his latest scope showed no more signs of precancer or erythematous patches.

Additionally, John has incorporated a daily intake of 400 mg of SAMe (a supplement that helps maintain a stable mood and supports both joint and liver health) to address depression that persisted for years, and he is pleased to report that it has now resolved.

Paraphrased testimonial from Henderson and Garcia's book:

Years ago, **Dr. Siegfried Ernst, M.D.** faced a cancer diagnosis that led to major surgery, resulting in the removal of his stomach. Two years later, the cancer recurred, and the recommended remedy was chemotherapy. However, given the limited hope for survival—typically less than a year for individuals with this type of cancer—Dr. Ernst opted against chemotherapy. Recognizing the ineffectiveness and detrimental impact on quality of life, he turned to Dr. Budwig and her formula for assistance.

Devotedly adhering to Dr. Budwig's formula, Dr. Ernst has experienced no cancer recurrence over the past fifteen years. Remarkably, he is now in perfect health and displays an energetic vigor uncommon for a man in his late seventies.

Take action now. To get started with your new dietary regimen, here are some essential steps to follow:

Make a list of the items you need to buy. Head to a store that stocks Nancy's cottage cheese and purchase enough for a week.

Place an order with Barlean's for flax oil. Ask for the 'cancer discount' while placing your order. Order six bottles to save on time and shipping costs.

Order/buy a good hand blender if you don't already have one.

Begin your new dietary regimen as soon as possible!

The next chapter discusses the *next big thing* you can do to get well.

CHAPTER 3

The Center and the Formula

Next, my research guided me to the **Hoxsey Bio Medical Center.**[1] The Center was initially brought to my attention by Ty and Charlene Bollinger, renowned for their work on the website The Truth About Cancer. Even before my diagnosis, one of their video series grabbed my attention, offering insight into alternative healing possibilities for cancer.

In Bollinger's The *Truth About Cancer*[2] documentary series A Global Quest, Ty recounted the story of how his father, Graham Bollinger, had been diagnosed with stomach cancer in 1996, and they tried to get him to the Center in Mexico. Still, his father had unfortunately died before they could get him there. Ty recounted how he was excited to take the video production team to the Center to learn more about the treatment. He interviewed the owner of the Center at the time, Liz Jonas, the sister of Mildred Nelson, who was Harry Hoxsey's (more about him in a minute) chief nurse. Mildred originally intended to "expose" Harry Hoxsey and his cancer center in Texas as a fraud. Instead, Mildred's mother, who had cancer, was treated with the formula and lived to be ninety-nine years old. Mildred had a change of heart and became Harry's head nurse. Harry passed the Hoxsey formula on to Mildred, who passed it on to her sister Liz, who became the new owner of the Center.

When my diagnosis came, I remembered this story. This recollection led me to the re-discovery of the Hoxsey Bio Medical Center. At the time, their website needed updating, but today, it is updated and refined, and offers an excellent summary of their services, what to expect, and even travel and hotel recommendations.

I delved into their history, which started in the late 1800s. According to the book *You Don't Have to Die* (now out of print) by Harry Hoxsey, Harry's great-grandfather, John Hoxsey, a horse breeder by trade, stumbled upon a revelation that would lead him to the creation of the Hoxsey formula. He observed that horses on the brink of succumbing to cancer tumors regained their health after consuming specific herbs found nearby. These herbs somehow helped the horses regain their health, and through experimentation, he distilled them into the first iteration of the Hoxsey formula.

The formula's potency was undeniable. Horses that were once doomed to die now stood as evidence of its effectiveness. News of this amazing formula spread among the equestrian community, and soon, horse owners from far and wide sought out Harry's great-grandfather and his remedy.

The formula got passed down through the generations until it ended up in the hands of Harry's father John (same name as the great-grandfather), when it was revised for use with humans.

The success of the Hoxsey Formula became widely known for treating cancer patients with more and more stories of healing. Celebrities and politicians, among others, sought help from the Hoxsey Bio Medical Center, which offered the formula. By 1962, seventeen clinics in the United States, one in each major city, were treating 12,000 cancer cases annually.

In 1964, a landmark lawsuit between Dr. Fishbine of the American Medical Association (AMA) and Dr. Harry Hoxsey culminated in Hoxsey's win, as **he proved the effectiveness of his herbal formulas in treating many cancers.** However, the FDA padlocked all seventeen clinics in operation immediately after, citing the use of unapproved medicines. The clinic then moved to Tijuana, Mexico, where it still operates.

Despite the controversy, the Center still stands as an alternative cancer treatment center for those seeking a different path, with a holistic approach and the guidance of licensed physicians.

For more on the history of the Hoxsey formula and clinic, see the book *Hoxsey Therapy: When Natural Cures for Cancer Became Illegal; The Autobiography of Harry Hoxsey, ND*; and *When Healing Becomes a Crime: The Amazing Story of the Hoxsey Cancer Clinics and the Return of Alternative Therapies* by Kenny Ausubel.

I reached out to the Center, and here is what I experienced: the process was pretty easy. I scheduled an appointment and made travel arrangements. Their website recommends where to stay overnight, etc., if that is what you decide to do. I live two hours from San Diego, so I drove there and stayed two nights. The appointment takes almost the whole day, so I opted to stay an extra night so that I didn't feel rushed or stressed about getting home. I stayed overnight at the Comfort Inn on the American side of the border. They have a special rate for those with appointments at the Center. Early in the morning of my appointment, a medical van (free with the Comfort Inn reservation) transported me and several others through a special medical entrance to Mexico, skipping the long lines of people crossing the border.

The staff and doctors welcomed me warmly and respectfully when I arrived at the Center. The backdrop was an upscale suburb of Tijuana, more evidence of the Center's commitment to providing dignified care. The day unfolded beginning with scans and blood work (although these are unnecessary if you provide your recent results from your doctors), consultations with the doctor, and a meeting with a nutritionist. Cancer can create a lot of fear and anxiety, so the Center also has counseling services available if you want to take advantage of this.

They instructed me to fast, so I was hungry by mid-morning, and I took advantage of their lovely little café and had breakfast while they worked on getting test results. Amidst the camaraderie of fellow patients, we shared stories of hope and healing.

After my final consult with the doctor and prescriptions in hand, I met with "Olga," picked up my Hoxsey formula, and paid my balance with a credit card. The balance of my herbal medications would be shipped from the States to my home in a few days. Prescriptions are tailored to each patient's particular situation. For example, they prescribed me an herbal formula for "Melanoma" in addition to the Hoxsey formula.

The pandemic prompted the Center to adapt, and I was able to have my six-month checkup with the physician remotely. If you are a new patient, I'm pretty sure they will want to see you, at least initially, in person. There may be exceptions; you should check with them on that. But as long as I remain cancer-free, I think they will offer remote sessions. I have one more session to go in a few months, and I believe I will go once a year, or perhaps not meet at all unless I show signs of cancer again. If that happened, I would call them in a heartbeat.

Expected Costs for Natural Treatments

In my case, my cancer diagnosis began with a stage IV diagnosis. My insurance covered my lung surgery, my CT scans, doctor visits, bloodwork, and immunotherapy (which we stopped). The Budwig

Diet recommended in Chapter 2 can fit into your regular grocery budget. The Hoxsey Bio Medical Center will tell you your cost may be around $1,500 to $1,800 for treatment and herbal medicines (which amounts to $250 to $300 per month)—my Hoxsey Treatment Center expenses, including doctor visits and herbal medications, average around $160 monthly. Your costs may vary depending on prescribed herbal medicines. With the potential of curing your cancer, these affordable alternatives empower you to delay costly conventional treatments, proving that healing doesn't have to come at an exorbitant price.

Patient Testimonials:

Christine Phillips
Diagnosis: Malignant Melanoma and Papillary Thyroid
Cancer Chemotherapy: Refused
Testimonial used with permission.

> After a biopsy of a mole on my jaw came back as melanoma, I had surgery immediately. Then, a wider excision of the original melanoma and the two sentinel lymph nodes came back positive for thyroid cancer. I was given a clean bill of health as to the melanoma, then had a thyroidectomy and was given one dose of a radioactive iodine tablet, which my endocrinologist told me would easily eradicate the thyroid cancer.
>
> Four months later, melanoma appeared above my collar bone, in my neck and armpit area, skull, chest wall, and thyroid lymph nodes.
>
> I was referred to one of the top cancer research hospitals in the country, where I was told the only hope they

could offer me was biochemotherapy, a treatment that would leave me hospitalized for two weeks out of every month, completely disabled for up to a year, and I was told that I may not even survive the treatment. If I did happen to survive, I was given a life expectancy of two to three years with multiple complications.

I arrived at the Bio Medical Center one week later. We saw Dr. Gutierrez for the first few visits and were so impressed with his kindness, knowledge, and expertise. He even found a lump in my armpit that two US doctors had missed. More spots appeared throughout the first year, but the doctors at Bio Medical Center were always on top of it, adjusting my treatment right away. Within three months, all of my labs and numbers were really good! I have felt great the entire time and been able to work full-time, with no side effects at all. I travel, hike, garden, and have an amazing quality of life! My PET scans and blood work have now come back totally clear for the last eighteen months, and no more cancer has been found.

Update from Christine in January 2024:

I know 100 percent that I would not be alive today, and thriving, if I did not go to Biomedical Center and get on your program. As of 2024, I am still doing great and am cancer-free.

You can watch dozens of YouTube videos of patient testimonials who were successfully treated at the Bio Medical Center here: https://youtube.com/playlist?list=UU0l_mGIFZ9gnNchXUAc_eRQ&si=MFvx4Pp7hvPku1V6

Or search YouTube for "Bonita Wellness" and watch their many video testimonials.

CHAPTER 4

Toxic-Free H2O: Navigating Fluoride and Chlorine Removal

The Dangers of Fluoride

Staying hydrated with fresh, pure water is critical to our overall health. I discovered the dangers of fluoride in our water supply many years ago, and I'm so grateful that I did! This chapter discusses those dangers and why you should filter out fluoride and chlorine from your drinking and bathing water.

Remembering those '80s toothpaste commercials is a trip down memory lane. You remember the Aquafresh ads, proudly touting fluoride as the unbeatable weapon against cavities. They had this special gel for minty-fresh breath, and fluoride was "clinically proven" to tackle cavities. Looking back, it's amusing to think we believed those claims.

Now, let's talk about fluoride—that seemingly innocent element that's practically everywhere. It's in our tap water, oral care products, and prescription drugs. It flows from our faucets, quenching our thirst and making its way into our everyday routines. But here's the kicker: this supposed dental hero might not be as friendly as it seems. Most municipal water supplies are swimming with fluoride, leading to water toxicity and potential consequences we never considered. It's not just our health on the line; this contamination impacts the well-being of millions.

In an alarming statement, The Truth About Cancer (TTAC) has reported that fluoride in our water has "led to the deaths of millions of Americans and weakened the immune systems of tens of millions more."[1] The very substance promoted as a safeguard for dental health is now raising concerns about its potential harm.

Evidence of the destructive influence of fluoride is not hard to find. Take, for instance, the Eyjafjallajoekull volcano eruption in 2010. The attention wasn't on the lava flows or the ash clouds but on the aftermath of fluoride poisoning that occurred. Volcanic ash, with a naturally occurring elevated concentration of soluble fluoride, can spread across extensive land areas following volcanic eruptions. An article by the BBC on April 19, 2010, gives a stark account of what happened, highlighting the devastating effects of fluoride on life in the area. After the eruption, nearby animals were severely harmed, and a sinister legacy was left behind.[2]

The problems with fluoride are not a new revelation. The disturbing use of fluoride was exposed decades ago when US Air Force Major George R. Jordan testified before the Un-American Activity Committee of Congress in the 1950s. Major Jordan's shocking testimony unveiled a dark truth—during his tenure as a USA-Soviet liaison officer in the 1930s, the Soviets openly admitted to using fluoride in the water supplies of their concentration camps. The purpose? To render the prisoners docile, subservient, and, perhaps most chillingly, deliberately less intelligent. The use of fluoride in our daily lives is shrouded in mystery, and recent revelations have cast a disturbing shadow over its history.

While many of us were raised to believe that fluoride in tooth-paste is a critical player in the fight against dental decay, the reality of its effects on children and adults may be far more alarming. Fluoride toothpaste has become a pervasive fixture in our daily oral hygiene routines, promoted as a protector of our pearly whites. However, the unintended consequences of fluoride toothpaste use have been well documented. Excessive fluoride exposure can lead to dental fluorosis, which discolors and damages teeth. In severe cases, dental fluorosis can result in enamel pitting and staining, impacting both the aesthetic and structural integrity of our teeth. It's essential to recognize that children are particularly vulnerable to these effects, as their developing teeth are more susceptible to the toxic potential of fluoride.

In his book, *Fluoride, The Aging Factor*, Dr. John Yiamouyiannis sounded a dire warning, emphasizing that fluoride is, in fact, a poison.[3] It's sobering to consider that fluoride has been employed as a pesticide for combating mice, rats, and various small pests, a testament to its toxic nature. Dr. Yiamouyiannis stressed the incredible strength of fluoride, stating that a quantity of only one one-hundredth of an ounce could be fatal for a ten-pound infant. In contrast, just one-tenth of an ounce could have the same deadly effect on a one-hundred-pound adult. In 1977, Dr. Dean Burk, who formerly headed the US National Cancer Institute's cell chemistry section, conducted epidemiological studies with Yiamouyiannis, revealing a deeply troubling reality. Their research indicated that **fluoridation was significantly correlated with approximately 10,000 cancer-related deaths each year.** The shocking conclusion was that fluoride was responsible for more human cancer cases, and at a faster rate, than any other chemical. In the past thirty years, more people have died from cancer-related to fluoridation than the total number of military deaths in the entire history of the United States, according to Dr. Yiamouyiannis.

A notable study conducted by the Harvard School of Dental Health in 2005 revealed a concerning connection between fluoride exposure and osteosarcoma, a rare and aggressive form of bone cancer, particularly among young boys. This discovery raises questions about the safety of fluoride present in dental products and water. Sodium fluoride, the chemical used for this purpose, can adversely affect our health beyond just dental health. It has been observed to hinder the activity of essential enzymes, paralyze white blood cells, and even break down collagen, which is important for our body's defense against diseases like cancer. In other words, fluoride poses a significant threat to our overall health. Over 500 peer-reviewed studies have confirmed the harmful effects of sodium fluoride, ranging from increased cancer risk to potential brain damage. The evidence challenges the belief that fluoride is safe and calls for a reevaluation of its widespread usage.

Fluoridated water has caused devastating consequences globally, with alarming stories emerging from India. In the village of Gaudiyan, well over half of the population has been affected by bone deformities, resulting in physical handicaps that afflict both children and adults. These defects manifest after children start consuming fluoridated water, causing crippling deformities in their hands and feet. These children were born healthy, but the fluoride in their drinking water has had a cruelly debilitating impact on their lives.[4]

One medical expert, Dr. Amit Shukla, a neurophysician, drew a direct link between the excessive fluoride content in drinking water and these disabilities. The key issue lies in the body's impaired ability to absorb dietary calcium due to the elevated fluoride levels in the water, ultimately leading to disabilities and deformities. The doctors in the Indian government have denied any association between fluoridation of drinking water and debilitating conditions despite evidence to the contrary. They have stubbornly refused to perform water tests, asserting that such examinations are "not necessary."

In Pavagada village, there is a concerning issue where children are struggling with blindness caused by lamellar congenital cataracts. This condition damages the eye lenses. After medical assessment, local doctors have identified two main factors contributing to the child blindness crisis: consanguineous marriages (those between close blood relatives) and a high "fluoride content" found in the local water supply.

The History of Fluoride in our Water Supply

The history of fluoride in our water supply is a disturbing story of how corporate interests, backdoor politics, and cunning public relations turned a toxic poison into a so-called "safe" component of our daily lives. In the early 1900s, the canning industry's rapid growth significantly increased aluminum manufacturing. Unfortunately, this produced a lot of toxic waste, including sodium fluoride. Disposing of this hazardous byproduct was expensive, which prompted the Aluminum Company of America's (ALCOA's) founder and major stockholder, Andrew Mellon, to devise a clever solution.

Mellon had a plan to become the Secretary of the Treasury, which gave him authority over the US Public Health Services (PHS). He used this strategic placement to prepare for a significant shift in the system. Gerald J. Cox, a scientist funded by ALCOA, made an unsupported claim that fluoride was good for dental health. In 1939, Cox suggested adding fluoride to the USA's water reservoirs.

This drastic decision was not made by a doctor, a dentist, or a legit-
imate researcher but by a scientist working for the nation's largest
fluoride producer.

During the early stages of adding fluoride to the water supply, the
American Dental Association and American Medical Association
protested against it. They urged Congress to stop this toxic practice.
"In the 1940s, countless studies proved conclusively that fluoride
is toxic, causes cancer, damages the immune system, causes brain
damage, and damages internal organs."[5] However, with the support
of the Military Industrial Complex, ALCOA classified the results
of all these studies to hide the adverse effects of fluoride.

In 1947, Oscar R. Ewing, a lawyer who had worked for ALCOA
for years, was chosen to lead the Federal Security Agency, which
gave him control over the PHS. Despite its toxicity, the organization
began a nationwide campaign during Ewing's tenure to add sodium
fluoride to water supplies. This initiative was promoted by Edwin
L. Bernays, a master of public relations known as the "Father of
Spin" and the nephew of Sigmund Freud.

Bernays was a pioneer in the application of his uncle's psycho-
logical theories to advertising and government propaganda. In his
book, *Propaganda*, he championed the notion of "scientific manip-
ulation of public opinion." He believed that a select few individuals
could secretly control the masses. Bernays' tactics involved claim-
ing favorable research findings without substantial evidence and
repeating these assertions until they became accepted truths. Any
detractors were promptly branded as lunatics, effectively muzzling
opposition.[6] In 1950, the government officially endorsed water
fluoridation, and today, nearly 73 percent of the nation's water

reservoirs are fluoridated, with almost 150,000 tons of sodium fluoride each year, despite its status as a hazardous waste product and the litany of health concerns it raises.[7]

What about Chlorine?

Adding chlorine to municipal water supplies is important to keep them clean from harmful bacteria and contaminants. However, filtering chlorine and fluoride from your drinking and bathing water is equally crucial. You can purchase good quality water filters that remove chlorine and fluoride. It is also important to use a showerhead filter that can filter out these toxins. Your skin, the largest organ in the body, can absorb these toxins while bathing, and inhaling chlorine vapors can harm your health.

Jon Barron, a health researcher and alternative medicine advocate, has expressed concerns about the presence of chlorine in drinking water. He suggests that the chlorine added to municipal water supplies for disinfection can adversely affect health. Barron is known for raising questions about the potential risks of chlorine exposure, primarily through drinking water and bathing or showering.

Some of his key points about chlorine in drinking water include:

Chlorine Disinfection Byproducts: Barron has pointed out that the reaction between chlorine and organic matter in water can lead to the formation of disinfection byproducts, such as trihalomethanes (THMs) and haloacetic acids (HAAs). These byproducts may have harmful health effects and are a subject of concern.

Respiratory and Skin Irritation: He suggests that the chlorine in tap water can vaporize during showering, potentially causing respiratory irritation. Additionally, exposure to chlorinated water during bathing or showering might be associated with skin dryness or irritation for some individuals.

Possible Carcinogenicity: Jon Barron raises the question of the potential carcinogenic effects of chlorine and its byproducts. While the evidence linking chlorine to cancer remains controversial, he emphasizes the importance of minimizing exposure.

Water Filtration: To address these concerns, Barron often recommends using water filtration systems to remove or reduce chlorine and its byproducts from drinking water.

Chapter Summary and What Can I Do?

In summation, the story of fluoride in our water supply illustrates the alarming reality that fluoride is essentially a hazardous waste by-product from industries such as aluminum, fertilizer, and nuclear energy. Instead of bearing the disposal costs for this hazardous waste, these industries have discovered a convenient avenue for their toxic by-products: selling them to municipalities for water fluoridation. This process essentially amounts to mass-medicating the entire population through our water supply. When examined closely, the implications of such an approach are deeply troubling, raising serious questions about the ethics and wisdom of exposing entire communities to these risks and toxic substances.

After learning about this concerning revelation, you might wonder what steps you can take to address it. The first and most important step is to ensure your water is free from harmful contaminants, specifically chlorine and fluoride. One option is to choose Arrowhead Mountain spring water from the San Bernardino Mountains in Southern California (I have it delivered to our home). If this is unavailable in your area, I recommend considering the Berkey Water Filter system (which we also use), which can be purchased through their website.[1] This system can have filters that eliminate chlorine, fluoride, and other impurities. Alternatively, you can check out an under-sink water filter that attaches to your cold-water valve and effectively removes these contaminants. Additionally, purchasing a shower head filter to remove chlorine and fluoride while bathing is important. Remember, the purity of the water you drink and use for daily activities is crucial to your overall health and well-being. And make sure to stay adequately hydrated!

CHAPTER 5

Chemotherapy: Is It a Cure or a Curse?

As mentioned earlier in this book, I consider myself lucky to have never faced the decision of whether or not to undergo chemotherapy. As a reminder, I attempted immunotherapy (a medical treatment that stimulates the body's immune system to target and combat diseases, particularly cancer) but had to stop due to an autoimmune reaction. At that point, my oncologist informed me that without further treatment, I likely had eight to ten months left to live. He also clarified that chemotherapy would not cure me but only delay the inevitable. We decided to wait until the next CT scan before considering any other treatments, and I began researching my options.

In this chapter we cover an interview where a doctor discusses some of the pros and cons of chemotherapy.

Interview with a Doctor

Dr. Irvin Sahni, M.D., stated in an interview with Ty Bollinger, author of *The Truth About Cancer* that discussing alternative or natural methods of curing cancer could lead to investigation and possible prosecution by the medical board. Oncologists are not incentivized to discuss such methods, and many may be afraid to bring up these alternative and natural treatments. Below is the transcript from the interview (with permission):[1,2]

Ty Bollinger: One could make the argument that chemotherapy is never needed in a sick body, couldn't they?

Dr. Sahni: Well, yes. And here's where I might diverge from you a little bit, from this line of thinking, and we talked about this before. In my opinion, chemotherapy is very different, depending on the type of cancer. So, if you look at, let's say—here's a really interesting comparison. If you look at gonad cancer . . . .

Ty Bollinger: Testicular, sure.

Dr. Sahni: Yeah, testicular cancer, seminoma, and you compare it to the female version of the gonads, which is the ovaries. If you look at patients who have testicular cancer, their survival rates with chemotherapy are 95 percent. So, I would certainly argue, in the case of seminoma, that particular chemotherapy, although it may be toxic, tends to be very successful. In the case of pancreatic cancer or ovarian cancer, the results are abysmal. And the five-year survival rate is somewhere in the order of a few percentage points. And so, in that case, yeah, I completely agree.

But there are some forms of cancer where I do believe chemo-therapy is a good option. Now if there were a natural way to treat that cancer, then absolutely. I've always argued in all the Quest Series that they are not necessarily telling people, and I know you're not telling people to abstain or avoid conventional treatments, what you're saying is there's other choices out there. And after reviewing natural means or alternative means and you want to go back and do those conventional treatments, maybe because it's seminoma versus ovarian cancer, then that's exactly what this is all about.

It's about education, information, and being self-empowered in making your own decisions based on the facts, not inserting your bias. But the problem is when you go to see an oncologist, at least as far as I know, they don't offer you those other opportunities. The menu is very short. The menu is typically three things—chemotherapy, radiation, and surgery.

And, if an oncologist wanted to discuss other alternative or natural means of curing your cancer, they would probably be investigated by the medical board and possibly even prosecuted in some cases, depending on the situation. Not only are they not incentivized to do it, but I think in a lot of cases, they are probably scared to even bring up some of these truths.

Ty Bollinger: Actually, we agree on that—the testicular cancer. There are a few rare cancers that the chemo does actually work on. I think my question was that it was really more intended to bring out the fact that people are not sick with cancer because they're shy on chemotherapy. So, the reason they're sick is not that they're chemotherapy-deficient. Not that there are certain cancers that chemo doesn't work on, like some non-Hodgkin's lymphoma, testicular cancer, and a few other cancers.

Dr. Sahni: Chemotherapy is not a vitamin. Chemotherapy is not a vitamin D or a vitamin C. If they were to correct their physiology, and they were to give their body the nutrition or abstain from the toxins that cause the cancer, they would actually solve the problem. If someone is exposed to a chemical that is known to cause cancer, they get cancer. They get chemotherapy, and let's say they get lucky, and they're successfully treated with chemotherapy, but then they go back and get exposed to that chemical again.

Well, guess what? They're going to have cancer again. The chemotherapy didn't fix that. The chemotherapy may have placated it, even if it worked, like we just said. And in some cases, there is only 3 percent success rate overall. The problem is not a deficiency of chemotherapy. The problem is some other outside factor that's causing them to be sick.

Ty Bollinger: That's definitely what I was trying to get to; that chemotherapy can be a very effective Band-Aid. Sometimes it can be a huge Band-Aid, and maybe it's a permanent Band-Aid, but it never really corrects that imbalance.

Dr. Sahni: I think a lot of people still believe—because I talk to patients all the time about this—and they really believe that the fact that they're going to get cancer is sort of preordained. It's in their genes. It's nothing they can do about that. They have no control over it.

They don't realize that by cleaning up their body or cleaning up the area in their life that's toxic that they absolutely cannot only prevent themselves from getting cancer but even cure or reverse cancer once they have it. I think that's still part of the big misconception. There's sort of bad luck. What can I do? What can I do but go to the doctor and get chemotherapy, radiation, or surgery?

The Side Effects of Chemotherapy

I am happy I never had to decide to try traditional chemotherapy because my natural treatments were effective soon enough that I did not have to discuss it with my oncologist.

Patients undergoing chemotherapy often struggle with a range of side effects, including fatigue, nausea, and hair loss. Chemotherapy can also weaken the immune system, making patients more vulnerable to infections. Other side effects may include anemia, changes in appetite, mouth sores, gastrointestinal issues, nerve damage, skin and nail changes, and potential fertility issues.

There have been concerns about the possibility of chemotherapy promoting the spread of cancer cells. Some studies suggest that, in some instances, chemotherapy may enhance the invasiveness of cancer cells and their ability to metastasize. This phenomenon needs to be better understood and remains a topic of ongoing research.

CHAPTER 6

Wellness Essentials: Other Key Elements for a Healthy Lifestyle

I strongly suggest incorporating the habits mentioned in the previous chapters to improve your overall health. This chapter discusses additional practices to increase your chances of avoiding or curing cancer. I highly recommend considering these habits for a healthier lifestyle.

Digestive Enzymes: Your Key to Optimal Wellness

I take digestive enzymes with every meal. These are in the form of a supplement taken with food. You can purchase them from any health food store or from a reliable online supplement store.

Dr. Edward Howell was a prominent researcher who emphasized the importance of digestive enzymes in maintaining good health. His work revolved around the concept that our diets have become enzyme-deficient

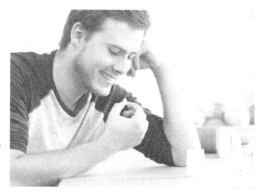

due to the prevalence of processed and cooked foods. He believed a lack of digestive enzymes in our diets could contribute to various health issues.

In his book *Enzyme Nutrition*, Dr. Howell explored the potential benefits of supplementing with digestive enzymes to support better digestion and overall well-being. His work inspired many to consider the role of enzymes in nutrition and health. His research underscores the significance of digestive enzymes in promoting optimal digestion and nutrient absorption.

Jon Barron, a health researcher and author, also highlights the significance of digestive enzymes in digestion and overall health. Barron's philosophy underscores the importance of digestive enzymes in breaking down food. Adequately digested food allows our bodies to absorb essential nutrients.

Barron suggests that due to factors like poor diet and aging, many individuals may have insufficient natural enzyme production, leading to digestive issues and a reduced ability to extract essential nutrients from their food. To address this, he often recommends digestive enzyme supplements to support proper digestion and alleviate related health concerns.

His work stresses the importance of these enzymes in helping the body efficiently process and utilize nutrients from the foods we consume, contributing to better overall health and well-being. Barron's approach to health and nutrition focuses attention on digestive enzymes as a key component of digestive health.

Taking digestive enzymes can assist our body in absorbing essential nutrients from the food we eat. It can also help us have regular bowel movements, which is crucial for detoxifying our system. Proper digestion, nutrient absorption, and detoxification are all critical factors in maintaining a healthy gut and overall well-being.

Given the prevalence of poor diets and sedentary lifestyles, enzyme supplements are necessary to ensure optimal health.

Probiotics: Your Gut's Best Friends

I take a probiotic every morning on an empty stomach. Having beneficial microorganisms in the gut is vital to your overall health. Jon Barron also emphasizes the importance of *probiotics* in maintaining overall health and well-being. He advocates for the use of probiotics as a way to support and restore the balance of beneficial microorganisms in the gut. Here are some key points that Jon Barron makes regarding the importance of probiotics:

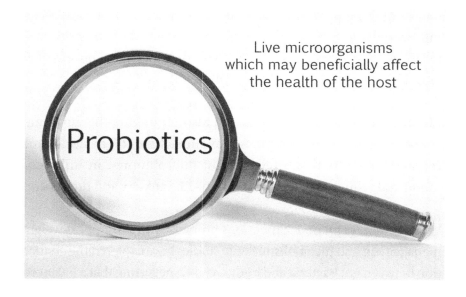

Live microorganisms which may beneficially affect the health of the host

Probiotics

Gut Health: Barron stresses the vital role of probiotics in promoting a healthy gut. Probiotics are live beneficial bacteria and yeasts that can help to restore and maintain the natural balance of microorganisms in the digestive system. A balanced gut microbiome is essential for proper digestion, nutrient absorption, and a robust immune system.

Digestive Health: He highlights the benefits of probiotics for individuals experiencing digestive issues, such as irritable bowel syndrome (IBS), constipation, or diarrhea. Probiotics help alleviate these symptoms and improve overall digestive health.

Immune Support: Jon Barron suggests that a significant portion of the immune system is located in the gut. Probiotics can enhance the immune response and help protect against infections and diseases. Maintaining a healthy gut microbiome is vital to immune system function.

Support During Antibiotic Use: He often discusses the importance of taking probiotics when using antibiotics. Antibiotics can kill harmful and beneficial bacteria, potentially disrupting the balance in the gut. Supplementing with probiotics during and after antibiotic treatment can help counteract this effect.

Mood and Mental Health: Barron also highlights the gut-brain connection and how probiotics may impact mental health. Some research suggests that a healthy gut microbiome can influence mood and reduce the risk of conditions like anxiety and depression.

Weight Management: He mentions probiotics might support weight management and metabolism. Some studies have explored the connection between gut bacteria and body weight, suggesting that a balanced gut microbiome may contribute to maintaining a healthy weight.

Food Allergies and Sensitivities: Barron notes that probiotics could help manage food allergies and sensitivities. They might contribute to the breakdown of certain compounds in food that could trigger allergic reactions or intolerances.

From Omnivore to Herbivore: Embracing Veganism

I became a vegan over many years, transitioning from a meat-based diet to a vegan one where all animal products, including meat, dairy, and eggs, are excluded. Before I was a vegan, I had many health problems, which led me to become a vegan. After

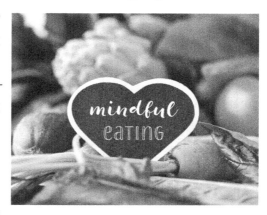

years of chronic illness, including constipation, frequent sinus infections, colds, or flu every year, I finally realized I was lactose intolerant and allergic to eggs! Being allergic to eggs also meant I would react every time I got a flu shot. Nowadays, I hardly ever get sick. I don't get flu shots anymore and haven't had the flu in many years.

Adopting a vegan lifestyle can bring about a host of health benefits. A plant-based diet is naturally low in saturated fats and cholesterol, making it an effective ally for heart health. It can help maintain an ideal body weight, reducing the risk of heart disease, high blood pressure, and type 2 diabetes. The abundance of fruits, vegetables, whole grains, and legumes provides essential nutrients, fiber, and antioxidants, which support overall vitality. Additionally, vegans often experience improved digestion and lower blood pressure, reducing the risk of certain cancers. Choosing a vegan diet promotes personal well-being and contributes to a healthier and more vibrant life. It's also great for the environment.

It's important to note that the health benefits of a vegan diet are maximized when it is well-planned to ensure adequate intake of essential nutrients, particularly **vitamin B12, vitamin D,** calcium, iron, **omega-3 fatty acids,** and protein.

Beyond the Root: Why Removing Root Canals Matters

I'm amazed at how little I had heard about the issue with root canals negatively impacting overall health until I read about it and did some research. The information presented here is something the American Dental Association (ADA) and mainstream medicine do not want you to know about.

Root canals have been a standard dental practice for years. I had a root canal many years ago. Hearing about ongoing concerns about their safety prompted me to investigate the potential risks. A recent DNA study by the Toxic Element Research Foundation (TERF) supports earlier research that indicates teeth that have been treated with a root canal may contain toxic bacteria linked to various diseases. Advanced DNA testing identified pathological bacteria in root canal teeth, surrounding bone, and non-healing extraction sites, highlighting the need for further research to address potential health risks associated with dental procedures.

Patients should be empowered to make informed decisions.

In the early twentieth century, Dr. Weston Price discovered a link between bacterial growth in root canals and disease transmission.[1] However, dental associations have suppressed this information. The ADA still maintains this stance without any supporting research, and dentists risk losing their licenses if they discuss the dangers of root canals.

TERF argues that anaerobic bacteria in and around root canals are highly toxic and can contribute to various diseases.[2] I find it alarming that while people are aware of the hazards of alcohol and tobacco, many remain unaware of the disease-producing bacteria in root canals. DNA analysis challenges the perception that root canals are sterile and the data advocates for informed choices.

Dr. Hal Huggins, representing TERF, has conducted over four decades of dental material toxicity research and presented groundbreaking data on influential diagnostic chemistries. Many autoimmune disease patients have shown improvement, suggesting that removing challenging bacteria can aid recovery. This data addresses dental mercury, nickel, aluminum, root canal, and cavitation-related ailments and may help restore lives and prevent disease.[3] TERF aims to inform global health professionals and raise awareness for informed decision-making.

The Link to Cancer

Adding another perspective, Bill Henderson and Carlos M. Garcia, MD, discuss the impact of dental toxins on cancer patients in their book, *Cancer-Free: Your Guide to Gentle, Non-Toxic Healing.* Dr. Garcia operates the Utopia Wellness Center clinic in Clearwater, Florida, where he claims to successfully treat various types and stages of cancer and other conditions daily. According to the authors, toxins from root canals are a significant source of dental toxins and, according to them, most definitely cause cancer. They criticize the ADA for denying this issue and recommend reading *Root Canal Cover-Up* by the late George Meinig, D.D.S., F.A.C.D., a respected dentist.

I had one root canal and decided that I wasn't going to take any chances and explored how to get it removed. Henderson and Garcia point out that it is tough to find dentists who understand this issue and will remove your root canals. Here's what I did: I told my dentist that I was experiencing pain and discomfort in the tooth/crown where the root canal was done (fortunately for me, it was one of my rear-most teeth). I told them, rather than repair it, please remove it altogether!

The doctor did not blink an eye; he removed it, and my dental insurance covered it. There is now one missing tooth in my mouth, and it has not affected my smile in any way, and I don't even notice it's gone (one less tooth to floss). One more thing off the checklist to keep cancer from returning!

You can find holistic dental clinics in the United States and elsewhere that remove your root canals, but they may be expensive. One early reader of my book made me aware of this more affordable clinic: the American Biodental Center in Tijuana, Mexico. They follow the Huggins Protocol, which Dr. Hal A. Huggins created. This protocol implements holistic dental practices, considering potential health risks associated with dental procedures and materials. Some critical components of the protocol include biocompatibility testing to assess how patients respond to dental materials, a focus on the safe removal of mercury amalgam fillings, nutritional support for detoxification, and an overall holistic approach that considers how oral health impacts overall well-being. The protocol generally discourages root canals and advocates for alternative treatment options.

If you want to explore this issue even further, you might consider watching the movie *Root Cause*, a documentary film released in 2019 that explores the potential health risks associated with root canal procedures in dentistry. The film, directed by Frazer Bailey, is presented as an investigative journey by the filmmaker, who questions the safety of root canals and their potential links to systemic health issues.

Root Cause features interviews with various health professionals, patients, and experts, including dentists, who express concerns about the impact of root canals on overall health. The documentary suggests root canals may contribute to chronic health problems and autoimmune diseases.[4]

Of course, the movie has received criticism from the ADA and other organizations who argue that the documentary may present a biased and controversial perspective on root canals. But in my opinion, root canals are not worth the risk, especially if you are dealing with cancer. My advice is to get rid of them!

Enhancing Wellness: The Benefits of Smart Supplementation

When it comes to vitamin, herbal, and mineral supplementation, it's a personal decision. I've been taking various supplements since I was a teenager. My grandmother, whom I affectionately called "Nana," taught me the importance of taking a high-quality multivitamin, and I've made it a habit to supplement ever since. Over the years, I've changed what I take, but it has remained a consistent part of my life. It's worth noting 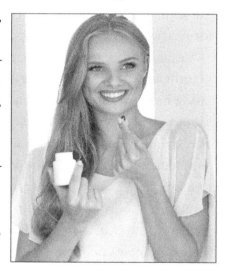 that even mainstream doctors are now stressing the importance of supplements, particularly vitamin D and vitamin B12. Nowadays, my typical blood work includes tests for those two supplements. If you're a vegan, it's essential to take vitamin B12, as it's naturally only found in meat products.

Vitamin B12

Vitamin B12 supplementation is essential for maintaining good health. This water-soluble vitamin plays a crucial role in keeping our nervous system healthy, aiding in the formation of red blood cells, and preventing anemia. It also supports DNA synthesis, which is essential for cell growth and division. Additionally, vitamin B12 promotes neurological health, helping to protect against conditions such as peripheral neuropathy.[5]

One of its most notable advantages is its ability to boost energy levels and combat fatigue, which is especially important for people with deficiencies. It also plays a significant role in maintaining cognitive function, contributing to memory and concentration. Additionally, this vitamin reduces homocysteine levels, a risk factor for heart disease, thereby supporting cardiovascular health.[6]

Vegans and vegetarians often rely on B12 supplements since it is mainly present in animal-based foods. In older adults, supplementation helps counteract age-related issues with B12 malabsorption. Vitamin B12 is crucial in maintaining DNA integrity, making it an effective agent in preventing cancer. With its diverse benefits, B12 supplementation ensures individuals have the necessary support to maintain a healthy and active lifestyle.

Natural sources of vitamin B12 include animal-based foods such as meat, fish, dairy products, and eggs. For those who follow a vegetarian or vegan diet, it can be challenging to obtain sufficient B12 from food alone, making supplementation a valuable option. It's important to note that B12 supplements come in various forms, including pills, sublingual tablets, and injections, and the choice may depend on specific health needs and conditions.

Vitamin D

It is crucial to **supplement with vitamin D** due to its many essential roles in maintaining overall health. This nutrient, also known as the "sunshine vitamin," is crucial for calcium absorption and bone health, which can help prevent conditions like osteoporosis. Moreover, vitamin D supports the immune system, reduces inflammation, and regulates mood, making it necessary for overall well-being.[7] Many people do not get enough sun exposure or dietary sources of vitamin D, which is why supplementation is often recommended. Insufficient vitamin D levels are linked to various health problems, such as a weakened immune system, increased susceptibility to infections, and a higher risk of chronic diseases.[7] Regular monitoring and appropriate supplementation help ensure that your body receives a sufficient amount of this vital nutrient.

Vitamin C

Vitamin C, which is also known as ascorbic acid, has a plethora of health benefits. It is famous for its antioxidant properties, which help safeguard your cells from damage caused by free radicals, reducing the risk of chronic diseases. This vital nutrient boosts your immune system, making it easier for your body to fight infections and recover from illnesses. Moreover, vitamin C is critical for collagen production, which contributes to maintaining healthy skin, blood vessels, and cartilage.[8]

Research has shown that sufficient vitamin C levels in your body can lower the risk of developing certain types of cancer.[9] To fully benefit from vitamin C, it is generally advised to include it in your daily diet. Fruits and vegetables such as oranges, strawberries, and bell peppers are excellent natural sources of this essential vitamin.

Proper pH Balance

Maintaining a healthy pH balance is crucial for good health, as Robert O. Young, Ph.D., and Shelley Redford Young emphasized in their book *The pH Miracle: Balance Your Diet, Reclaim Your Health.*

The authors highlight the association between acidity and cancer, explaining that cancer thrives in an acidic environment but diminishes in non-acidic conditions. According to the authors, cancer cells originate from once-healthy cells that dietary and metabolic acids have corrupted. The higher the acidity levels in the body, the greater the risk of developing cancerous tissue.[10]

The authors explain that healthy cells prefer a pH range of 7.3 to 11, thriving in mildly to highly alkaline fluids while being intolerant to mild acidity. Cancerous cells, on the other hand, thrive in an acidic pH of 5.5. These cells become dormant at a pH slightly above 7.365 and either revert to microzyma or perish at a pH of 8.5, while healthy cells flourish in an alkaline environment.[10]

I used to take barley powder from Green Supreme to make my body more alkaline. However, I stopped because I was concerned that it might interfere with the Hoxsey formula. Now that I am cancer-free, I have resumed taking the barley powder. If you use the Hoxsey formula, ask the Hoxsey Center if making your body more alkaline could interfere with it. If not, I highly recommend adding this supplement to your health regimen. Additionally, I believe that Green Supreme offers a 'cancer discount.'

Trim Your Sugar Intake

High sugar consumption is associated with an increased risk of cancer due to several mechanisms. Firstly, it can lead to obesity, a known risk factor for various cancer types. Additionally, sugar intake can cause insulin resistance, increasing insulin and IGF-1 production, both linked to cancer. It also promotes inflammation, potentially damaging DNA and aiding cancer growth. High-sugar diets can alter gut microbiota and promote the production of free radicals that can damage DNA.[11,12,13,14] Reducing cancer risk involves a balanced diet, limiting added sugars, emphasizing whole foods, maintaining a healthy weight, and staying active.

Meditation

I enjoy meditating as it helps me clear my thoughts and remain focused on the present moment, as Eckhart Tolle (author of *The Power of Now*) teaches us. I can avoid dwelling on the past or wor- 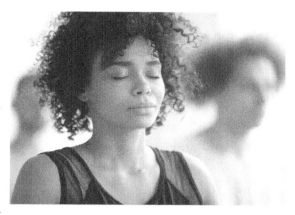 rying about the future by being fully present. Practicing meditation daily allows me to handle better any stressful situations that may arise throughout the day.

The centuries-old practice of meditation offers numerous benefits for physical, mental, and emotional well-being. Its ability to reduce stress is the most important benefit, as regular practice has been linked to lower levels of the stress hormone cortisol. Meditation also improves cognitive abilities such as focus, concentration, and overall mental performance. It promotes emotional stability and resilience, reducing symptoms of anxiety and depression. Additionally, calming the mind and reducing stress through meditation enhances sleep quality.[15,16,17,18] Meditation increases awareness of physical sensations and promotes attunement to the body by encouraging a stronger mind-body connection. It also alters pain perception and increases tolerance, leading to better pain management. Moreover, it facilitates personal growth and improved decision-making by fostering self-awareness through introspection. Its positive impact on cardiovascular health is evident in studies linking it to lower blood pressure.[19] Certain meditation techniques, such as loving-kindness meditation, encourage increased compassion and empathy towards oneself and others. Meditation significantly enhances mental health by promoting clarity, emotional stability, and cognitive function. It can help improve overall well-being and contribute to a healthier mind and body.

Yoga

My husband and I like to do yoga for stretching and relaxing. Yoga is a comprehensive practice that offers numerous benefits to the body and mind. Physically, yoga improves flexibility, strength, and balance 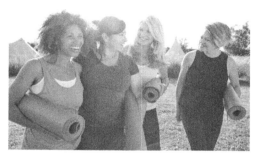 through various poses and stretches. It also encourages proper posture and body awareness, which can help prevent injuries.

Beyond its physical aspects, yoga is widely recognized for its stress-relieving properties. Combining controlled breathing, meditation, and mindful movement helps reduce cortisol levels and induces a sense of calm. Regular practice can improve mental focus, enhance emotional well-being, and alleviate symptoms of anxiety and depression.[20] Additionally, the emphasis on mindfulness fosters a deeper connection between the mind and body, promoting overall holistic health.

A Natural Prescription:
Exercise and Nature for Optimal Health

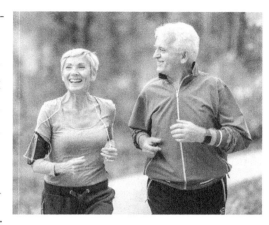

I maintain a regular exercise routine that includes weightlifting at the gym three times a week, using my at-home elliptical once or twice weekly, and taking long walks on the other days. When the weather allows, I enjoy hiking on trails outdoors. During the hot summer months, I purchase a summer pass for the Palm Springs Aerial Tramway, which takes me to the mountain station of San Jacinto State Park. This area offers miles of forested hiking trails and a temperature up to 30 degrees cooler than the hot desert floor where I live.

Benefits of Exercise

Regular exercise has numerous benefits that positively affect both physical and mental well-being. Firstly, it helps maintain a healthy weight by burning calories and promoting efficient metabolism. Exercise is also vital in improving cardiovascular health, reducing the risk of heart disease by enhancing blood circulation and lowering blood pressure. Physical activity also strengthens muscles and bones, leading to better overall physical fitness.[21]

Regular exercise not only has physical benefits but also profoundly affects mental health. It releases endorphins, which are often referred to as "feel-good" hormones. These hormones can alleviate stress, anxiety, and depression. Moreover, exercise enhances cognitive function, improving memory and concentration. Additionally, it promotes better sleep quality, which is crucial for overall health and well-being.

Regular physical activity has been shown to reduce the risk of chronic diseases like diabetes and cancer. It also strengthens the immune system and can help prevent illnesses.[21] Moreover, exercise is a great way to socialize, either by joining a group fitness class or a team sport, which can contribute to a sense of community and emotional well-being. By making exercise a part of your routine, you can take a holistic approach to achieving and maintaining optimal health.

Benefits of Being in Nature

Spending time in natural surroundings has numerous benefits for physical, mental, and emotional well-being. Firstly, studies have

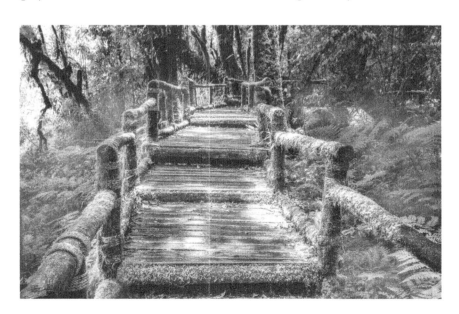

shown that being in nature can help reduce stress levels. The natural sights and sounds of trees, water, and birdsong are calming, promoting relaxation and lowering cortisol levels.[22]

Spending time in nature can lead to increased physical activity, as individuals engage in outdoor activities such as hiking, biking, or simply walking in a park. These activities can contribute to better fitness and cardiovascular health. Additionally, exposure to sunlight during outdoor activities can promote vitamin D production, which is essential for bone health and immune function.

Nature has a beneficial effect on mental health, relieving symptoms of anxiety and depression. It allows individuals to take a break from daily life's demands, helping them clear their minds and gain a fresh perspective. Nature is also linked to improved creativity and cognitive function.

Connecting with nature can inspire a profound sense of wonder and admiration for the world, which in turn cultivates mindfulness and gratitude. It encourages a deeper connection with the environment and a sense of interconnectedness. Ultimately, spending time in nature provides a holistic and rejuvenating experience that contributes to a healthier and more balanced life.

Combining regular exercise with outdoor activities in natural settings can amplify physical and mental health benefits. Whether it's a leisurely walk in the park, a hike in the mountains, or participating in outdoor sports, incorporating nature into your exercise routine can enhance overall well-being and provide a refreshing change of scenery from the demands of daily life.

Cultivate Positive Emotions

As I alluded to in the chapter on the emotions that come with a cancer diagnosis, keeping a positive outlook is really important.

Positive emotions offer a myriad of benefits that can significantly contribute to overall well-being:

♦ They play a pivotal role in promoting mental health by reducing symptoms of anxiety and depression which naturally come with a cancer diagnosis, fostering resilience, and aiding in stress management.

♦ Positive emotions have tangible effects on your physical health, including lower cortisol levels, improved immune function, and enhanced cardiovascular health.[23] These emotions also contribute to increased resilience, which can help you to navigate challenges with optimism and a constructive mindset.

♦ Positive emotions can positively impact your relationships by facilitating better communication, cooperation, and empathy.

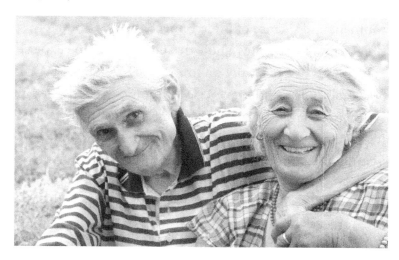

They are also linked to heightened creativity and improved problem-solving abilities, fostering innovation and cognitive flexibility. Positive emotions can help you with motivation and productivity, which can increase your engagement and efficiency. There are even associations between a positive outlook and increased longevity, as healthier lifestyle choices often accompany positive emotions. Moreover, positive emotions can help you with effective coping strategies and balanced decision-making, leading to greater life satisfaction and happiness. While acknowledging the natural ebb and flow of positive and negative emotions, actively cultivating positivity in daily life can yield you enduring benefits for overall well-being.

CHAPTER 7

The Next Steps are Yours

You stayed with me as I told you the story of my diagnosis and then through to the joyful finale where I lived to tell it. I'm six years cancer-free. Are you ready to begin your own healing journey?

Together, we relived the frightening diagnosis I received that shook me to the core of my being. Hospice workers were assigned to me and my family and told us they would do everything they could to keep me comfortable and as stress-free as possible as I worked my way through the weeks and months ahead. They thought I was going to die shortly after they met with me. My doctors did, too.

I recount how I decided **not to give up on myself** and moved forward with the research that ultimately saved my life.

I explained how I believe that **everything happens for a reason**, including finding things that would make me well and authoring this book so you, too, could have a fighting chance to beat cancer.

We reviewed the two things that contributed the most to my survival: the Budwig Diet and the Bio Medical Center and their life-saving natural remedies. We discussed how both are controversial among mainstream medical professionals, but not all. Many doctors and alternative treatment centers have successfully treated

their patients with these methods, and many thousands have testified to their healing from these treatments over the years.

I pointed out that although these two treatments are a mighty
force all their own, they are not all you can do to improve your
chances of surviving cancer.

We reviewed the importance of purifying your drinking and
bathing water of chlorine and fluoride, how and why both ended
up in our water supply, and why getting rid of them is essential.

I emphasized the importance of taking a digestive enzyme supplement with every meal and taking a probiotic daily, which will
help you stay regular and assist your body in eliminating toxins.

And don't forget how important it is to eliminate the mistakes
of root canals! We reviewed the medical reasons you must try to
eliminate them and some strategies for doing that. We reviewed
that some doctors assert that root canals are almost certainly a
significant source of cancer.

Finally, we reviewed several other important things you can
do to help improve your odds. We discussed everything from
regular exercise and getting out in nature to meditation, yoga,
a positive attitude, veganism, supplementation, and a regular
night's restful sleep.

In January 2024, as I was wrapping up the manuscript for my
book, I traveled to Amsterdam and then took a two-hour train and
a taxi ride to a serene retreat center called New Eden on a tranquil
forested land. The retreat focused on the theme of "Thriving in
Tribe." The weekend, co-hosted by Christian Pankhurst and his
business partner Sumir, emphasized the importance of community
or tribe and how together we can heal and thrive with the support
of others rather than trying to do it alone. Christian would say that
this is how we are meant to be—in community. This was the way

for thousands of years. Only recently have we become isolated and individualized. Getting back to community and tribe is essential to our thriving and healing as a species. You and I are now part of the same tribe/community of people seeking natural healing from cancer.

Don't give up on yourself! We are all in this together, and you have my, and many others, support. You can do this! You are not alone.

With much love and respect for your journey, William.

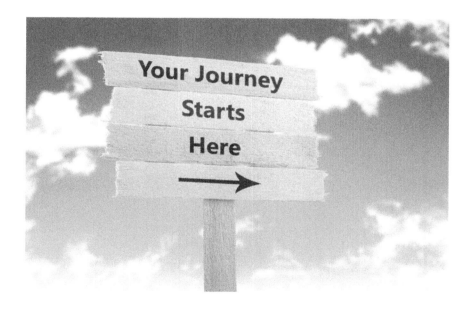

Endnotes

Chapter 2

1   "Complementary Cancer Support Clinic in Spain." Budwig Center, January 26, 2024. https://budwigcenter.com/.

2   Bill Henderson, and Carlos M. Garcia. *Cancer-free: Your guide to gentle, non-toxic healing.* Bradenton, FL: Booklocker.com, 2014.

3   "Budwig Center Client Testimonials—Cancer Survivor Stories." Budwig Center, January 22, 2024. https://budwigcenter.com/testimonials/.

Chapter 3

1   "Hoxsey Bio Medical Center: Alternative Cancer Treatment in Tijuana, Mexico." Hoxsey, August 24, 2023. https://www.hoxsey-biomedical.com/.

2   "The Latest Cancer-Fighting News." The Truth About Cancer. Accessed March 4, 2024. https://thetruthaboutcancer.com/.

Chapter 4

1   "Berkey Water Filter Systems—Replacement Filters & Accessories." My Berkey. Accessed March 4, 2024. http://www.myberkey.com/.

Chapter 5

1   Ty Bollinger, "Fluoride-Drinking Ourselves to Death?" The Truth About Cancer, August 9, 2022. https://thetruthaboutcancer.

com/fluoride-drinking-ourselves-to-death/?utm_campaign=m-mmm&utm_medium=social&utm_source=fb-ttac&utm_content=fluoride-drinking-ourselves-to-death&a_aid=59c13831797bc.

2   Unknown. "Toxic Ash Threatens Iceland Animals." BBC News, April 19, 2010. http://news.bbc.co.uk/2/hi/europe/8629241.stm.

3   John Yiamouyiannis, *Fluoride, the aging factor: How to recognize and avoid the devastating effects of flouride,* (Delaware, OH: Health Action Press, 1993).

4,5,6 Ty Bollinger, "Fluoride-Drinking Ourselves to Death?" The Truth About Cancer, August 9, 2022. https://thetruthaboutcancer. com/fluoride-drinking-ourselves-to-death/?utm_campaign=m-mmm&utm_medium=social&utm_source=fb-ttac&utm_content=fluoride-drinking-ourselves-to-death&a_aid=59c13831797bc.

7   Foundation, United Health. "Water Fluoridation in United States." America's Health Rankings. Accessed March 1, 2024. https://www. americashealthrankings.org/explore/measures/water_fluoridation.

Chapter 5

1   Ty Bollinger, and Dr Irvin Sahni. "Does Chemotherapy Work? (Video)." The Truth About Cancer, June 24, 2019. https://thetruthaboutcancer.com/does-chemotherapy-work-video/.

2   Permissions to quote *The Truth About Cancer* website obtained via email from Eric, Customer Service Representative, 11/3/23.

Chapter 6

1   American Biodental. *Root Canals Contain Toxic Bacteria.* Tijuana, MX: American BioDental Center, 2022. https://americanbiodental.com/brochures/biodental/root-c--plain-2022.pdf.

2,3   Ibid.

4   *Root Cause*, 2019. https://watch.plex.tv/movie/root-cause.

5   Poppy O. Smith, Ryan P Trueman, Rebecca Powell, Holly Gregory, James B Phillips, Patrizia Bohnhorst, and Melissa LD Rayner, "Longdom Publishing SL: Open Access Journals." Longdom, March 15, 2023. https://www.longdom.org/open-access/exploring-the-effect-of-vitamins-b1-b6-and-b12-on-neurite-regeneration-using-a-3d-coculture-model-of-neurodegeneration-100249.html.

6   Michael Atsushi Kimura, Ryuta Kinnno, and Kenjiro Ono. "Effects of Vitamin B12 on Cognitive Function in Elderly Patients." Alzheimer's Association, 2021. https://alz-journals.onlinelibrary.wiley.com/doi/abs/10.1002/alz.055458.

7   Shahzadi Devje, "Vitamin D: Benefits, Sources, Deficiencies." Healthline, February 6, 2023. https://www.healthline.com/health/food-nutrition/benefits-vitamin-d.

8   Ryan Raman, "7 Impressive Benefits of Vitamin C Supplements." Healthline, February 19, 2020. https://www.healthline.com/nutrition/vitamin-c-benefits#The-bottom-line.

9   Lewis Cantley, and Jihye Yun. "Intravenous High-Dose Vitamin C in Cancer Therapy." National Cancer Institute, 2020. https://www.cancer.gov/research/key-initiatives/ras/news-events/dialogue-blog/2020/yun-cantley-vitamin-c.

10   Robert O. Young, and Shelley Redfor Young. *The PH miracle: Balance your diet, reclaim your health.* New York: Warner Books., 2010.

11   Paresh Dandona, Ahmad Alijada, and Arindam Bandyopadhyay. "Inflammation: The Link between Insulin Resistance, Obesity and Diabetes." Trends in Immunology, 2023. http://www.cell.com/trends/immunology/abstract/S1471-4906(03)00336-3.

12   Karina Garcia, Gonçalo Ferreira, Flávio Reis, and Sofia Viana. "Impact of Dietary Sugars on Gut Microbiota and Metabolic

Health." MDPI, October 28, 2022. https://www.mdpi.com/2673-4540/3/4/42.

13   CDC. "Obesity and Cancer." Centers for Disease Control and Prevention, August 9, 2023. https://www.cdc.gov/cancer/obesity/index.htm.

14   Francesca Marciano, and Pietro Vajro. "Oxidative Stress and Gut Microbiota." ScienceDirect, June 9, 2017. https://www.sciencedirect.com/science/article/abs/pii/B9780128053775000084.

15   Andy Fell, "Mindfulness from Meditation Associated with Lower Stress Hormone." UC Davis, January 24, 2016. https://www.ucdavis.edu/news/mindfulness-meditation-associated-lower-stress-hormone.

16   Peter Malinowski, and Liliana Shalamanova. "Meditation and Cognitive Ageing: The Role of Mindfulness Meditation in Building Cognitive Reserve—Journal of Cognitive Enhancement." SpringerLink, April 12, 2017. https://link.springer.com/article/10.1007/s41465-017-0022-7.

17   Ran Wu, Lin-Lin Liu, Xing-Hua Liu, and Chun-Lei Jiang. "Brief Mindfulness Meditation Improves Emotion Processing." Frontiers, September 24, 2019. https://www.frontiersin.org/journals/neuroscience/articles/10.3389/fnins.2019.01074/full.

18   Danielle Pacheco, and Dr. Anis Rehman. "Meditation and Sleep." Sleep Foundation, February 26, 2024. https://www.sleepfoundation.org/meditation-for-sleep.

19   Harvard Health. "Meditation and a Relaxation Technique to Lower Blood Pressure." Harvard Health, July 18, 2023. https://www.health.harvard.edu/heart-health/meditation-and-a-relaxation-technique-to-lower-blood-pressure.

20   J Thirthalli, G H Naveen, M G Rao, S Varambally, R Christopher, and B N Gangadhar. "Cortisol and Antidepressant Effects of Yoga." Indian journal of psychiatry, July 2013. https://www.ncbi.nlm.nih.gov/pmc/articles/PMC3768222/.

21   "Physical Activity for a Healthy Weight." Centers for Disease
      Control and Prevention, April 26, 2023. https://www.cdc.gov/
      healthyweight/physical_activity/index.html.

22   Jim Robbins, "Ecopsychology: How Immersion in Nature Bene-
      fits Your Health." Yale E360, 2020. https://e360.yale.edu/features/
      ecopsychology-how-immersion-in-nature-benefits-your-health.

23   Nancy L. Sin, "The Protective Role of Positive Well-Being in Car-
      diovascular Disease: Review of Current Evidence, Mechanisms,
      and Clinical Implications." Current cardiology reports, November
      2016. https://www.ncbi.nlm.nih.gov/pmc/articles/PMC5060088/.

      "Barley Grass for Healthy Human Bodies." Green Supreme, March
      4, 2024. https://greensupreme.net/.

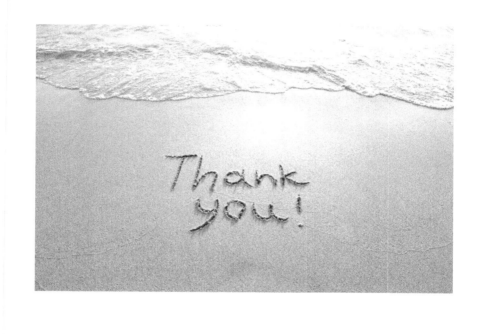

Acknowledgments

A special thank you to my "early readers" who read my transcript and gave me great suggestions on how to improve my book: Linda Bumpas, Dr. Robin Hallquist, MD, Jason Hardman, Stuart Huggins, Jaana Lehtola, Raymond Meyer, Wendy Colby Miller, Julie Notaro, Nan Papenhausen, and Phyllis Winters.

I also want to express my gratitude to Ty and Charlene Bollinger, who are behind *The Truth About Cancer* video series, for their assistance in finding solutions that helped me overcome cancer. I am also thankful to Dean Graziosi and Tony Robbins for inspiring me and pushing me to take my first steps towards authoring my book (through their 2023 Launchpad training program). Finally, I would like to thank Jack Canfield and Steve Harrison for their invaluable programs that equipped me with the necessary knowledge and skills to launch my book as a new author.

About the Author

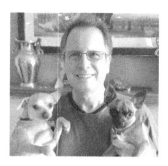

"An ordinary guy with an extraordinary story."

William Hudson, a stage IV cancer survivor, is a retired IT professional in higher education. He graduated magna cum laude from Pepperdine University in Malibu, California, earning a Bachelor of Science degree in Business Administration. William spent most of his career in higher education information technology at Pepperdine University and the University of Redlands. He spent a few years in the corporate realm as a higher education technology consultant and project manager at a 'big four' accounting firm and higher education software provider in San Francisco.

Besides his professional and writing pursuits, William enjoys exploring the scenic trails surrounding Palm Springs throughout the year. San Jacinto State Park is a favorite destination for his hiking adventures, especially during the summer when the elevation brings cooler temperatures than the scorching desert floor. At home near Palm Springs, William shares his life with his husband, two chihuahuas, two cats, and koi fish, creating a loving and fun environment.

Now in retirement and living in the beautiful southern California desert near Palm Springs, William fulfills his lifelong dream of writing and sharing his experiences and knowledge through the written word.

WilliamHudson.org

Made in United States
North Haven, CT
28 June 2024

54170976R00061